This book has been published in association with the Christian Evidence Society. The Society has existed since 1870 to present the fundamental truths of Christianity to enquirers. Its address is:

1 Little Cloister
Westminster Abbey
London
SW1P 3PL

Other titles in the series:

Why God?
Why Pray?
Why Belief?
Why Suffering?
Finding God in Bereavement
Finding God in Illness
Finding God in Marriage Breakdown

Finding God in Later Life

William Purcell

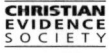

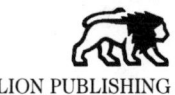

LION PUBLISHING

Copyright © 1997 William Purcell
The author asserts the moral right to be identified as the
author of this work

This edition published in 1997 by Lion Publishing plc Sandy
Lane West, Oxford, England
ISBN 0 7459 3718 7

Albatross Books Pty Ltd PO Box 320, Sutherland, NSW 2232,
Australia
ISBN 0 7324 1593 4

First edition 1997
10 9 8 7 6 5 4 3 2 1 0

All rights reserved
A catalogue record for this book is
available from the British Library
Printed and bound in India by Ajanta

Men are like wine:
some turn to vinegar,
but the best improve with age.

Pope John xxiii

Finding God in later life

The later years of life are a good time for trying to make a new life. 'Later years' can, of course, mean anything. We are always as old as we feel. Nowadays, with large numbers retiring annually and many living far longer than was once the case, the challenge to make a new start is all the greater, because there are going to be more years to use meaningfully. Changing patterns of employment affect this matter, too. Many people are asked to take early retirement and find themselves with virtually another life before them. This, as many have found, needs thinking about.

A useful first step in this thinking is to get rid of the old idea of retirement as something with geriatric overtones. That no longer fits the modern reality, when people can find themselves finished with full-time jobs in their early fifties. But, clearly, all of life has to be lived fully, not just the nine-to-five part of it that came at the beginning. The end of that beginning can, with planning, bring benefits.

There is no need at all to accept the dictionary definition of retirement as 'to withdraw, go away, retreat, seek seclusion, recede, go to bed, become recluse, be incommunicative or unsocial'! On the contrary, among the benefits of retirement may be the first rich experience of personal freedom to choose what is to be done with a new life. This presents a challenge as we face the need to advance, to go forward into a new way of living. It can involve some interesting re-adjustments. For one thing, it can lead to a change in the standard of values by which we live, so that those which were once held to be important, like material success, become downgraded, while very different things, such as learning new skills, developing new interests, and being of service to other people, especially those in need, become upgraded.

A typical figure in today's scene could be someone who has just left full-time employment. Pension, maybe with severance pay in the case of an early retirement, is perhaps not too bad. The heart of the matter is, however, that there are a lot of years left to live. It may seem a rather daunting prospect. It can be very helpful to sort the whole business out into some sort of order.

Experience suggests that there are four useful steps to take. The *first* is to get rid of any undue pre-occupation with the past—things as they were, things as they might have been. Putting all that behind makes room for a new future. The *second* is to explore positive ways—and there are many—of filling that future with meaningful activity. The *third* is to realize our limitations frankly, including physical ones, bearing in mind that by the time these new challenges reach us, we are not likely to be as youthful and vigorous as was once the case. In other words, cut the new suit according to the cloth available. *Lastly*—and for many this may be a new development altogether—it is deeply rewarding to give some time to cultivating the inner life of mind and spirit, by quiet, by study, and by giving some thought to what life is all about, how it can be lived with dignity and, for that matter, what may lie beyond it.

Getting rid of the past

This is so important that it needs firm handling. To keep thinking of yesterday is always a temptation, and many there are who fall for it. People like doctors and clergy, whose work takes them into counselling situations, speak of this as a frequent cause of unhappiness among older folk, sometimes causing actual physical ills. It makes living in the present more difficult, for one thing. After all, tomorrow is a possibility, yesterday is a memory; only today is a reality. Therefore to live in today, making the most of it, is the only sensible attitude. Brooding on what we have been is no good at all.

There was a good example of this in one of Alan Bennett's plays, *Sunset across the Bay*, where there was a man who had been a factory foreman and was proud of it. Retired to the seaside, and having given no thought to what that might involve, he found himself lost in a wasteland where there was nothing to do but continue to think of the past and of what he had been. He did not last long, and his wife soon joined the numerous ranks of widows there. If we are to overcome any temptation of the sort to which he fell victim, brooding on what we have been in terms of status, it helps to realize how natural it is and at the same time how unnecessary. It is natural because so many of us have lived in a lifestyle where climbing the ladder is important. It is futile because it doesn't matter any more, if indeed it ever did.

Another aspect of getting rid of the past involves abandoning some of the mental attitudes that might have seemed natural enough in the full tide of life. Then, it was normal to assume we were here forever, without giving much thought to the matter. But now, when trying to fashion a new sort of life, it matters that we should manage to cast off old attitudes and look out on life with new eyes. The truth is that we are, and always have been, creatures of the moment, and none of us can know how much more of life we are likely to have, whatever statistics may say. In fact we are all rather like people in a departure lounge at Heathrow waiting for their flight to be called.

To grasp hold of such basic truths is part of the new deal which comes with a new life in later years. One wise writer called this attitude the secret of successful retirement, whenever it comes, early or late. He also added as desirables reasonable physical health, an adequate income, congenial associates and neighbours and, very important, a sense of purpose in living. That last one is perhaps the key to the whole thing. Purpose, motive in being, whatever we like to call it is, like oxygen to the lungs, an essential. So the discovery of it is truly a big element in shaping a new life, going down new paths, expanding horizons. These are of the essence. That same writer on retirement added, 'The aim is not to find an elixir of youth, or to seek to turn back the clock; but to enable people who have reached later years to find opportunities of fulfilling themselves with dignity, to the benefit of themselves and others.' What it amounts to is the second of those useful steps towards a new life mentioned earlier—filling the future with meaningful activity.

Filling the future

Here are several case histories of people who have done just that. All were interviewed within the last few years. The first had been editor of a county newspaper. He said, 'At first I had a feeling of guilt about not going off to work in the morning. That lasted about a fortnight. After that I found my time was occupied with jobs that might once have seemed humble, but were really just as useful as many of those I had been doing. There were two things that worried me: one was health, the other was money. Both proved groundless. Relieved of the worries and tensions of a demanding job, my health improved noticeably. I lost a stone in weight, because instead of sitting at a desk all day I was now out and about. As for money, I seem to have more in my pocket than before, maybe because I live much more simply. This in spite of a substantial drop in income. This new life has riches to offer. There is freedom of movement, power to choose how to spend one's time, and, above all, possession of time itself. Opportunities to be useful soon presented themselves.'

After looking around he found a suitable use for his time and talents by becoming editor of his local diocesan magazine. He added, 'One is one's own master, perhaps for the first time ever, since most of us live in some kind of bondage, in childhood to parents, in youth to school, in working life to the job and one's employers. But now that is cast off, and there is a life to be lived according to bent and inclination.'

Next, the experience of a rather older man who had spent the whole of his working life in the Post Office. 'When I came to retire,' he said, 'I felt this was the opportunity to pursue, in my own time and ways, some of the many interests I had always had. And then others came along, and they fill my life now. I think a great deal of the success of my retirement is based on the fact that I already had things I wanted to do and was therefore ready for it. I had always felt that retirement needed careful preparation. I had seen too many people who had failed to do so, and who sort of walked out into a void when their jobs finished. Some seemed just to die away, in a few cases literally.'

This man's case contrasts strongly with that of another man I met about the same time. He had held an important position as head of an engineering concern and had lived always entirely absorbed in his work, taking a pride, indeed, in his total devotion to it. Retirement hit him hard, and he gave the impression of being a deeply unhappy person, without having any idea of why he was so. Something else which the former Post Office man said could have given him a clue: 'I looked forward to retirement as something promising on the horizon, and now I have developed further interests I once had in embryo. For instance, I was always interested in local history; now I am secretary of my Local History Society. In addition, and on another line, I teach a bit of Art Appreciation—another of my earlier interests—in a Retirement Association. Strangely, I seem to have little time for myself.'

Asked to comment on the biblical theme, 'Happiness lies more in giving than in receiving', he added the deeply significant words: 'That's true. Forgetfulness of yourself is the surest way out of frustration. Show me a selfish man and I'll show you a bored one.'

Two further cases show a deep truth of another kind; that time spent in the service of others, in addition to the pursuit of personal interests, however worthy, can be the most rewarding of all. One is the rather formidable woman who had been a business executive. She said, 'I have had ten happy years after a fairly early retirement. Then I started voluntary work with a Citizen's Advice Bureau. What a lot that has taught me about how the other side of the world lives, a side very different from what I had been used to! I have learnt to be concerned with people carrying intolerable burdens, with the unlucky, with the inadequate who simply can't cope with the world. I hope I have helped to ease some of their problems.' It had been, she said, an unexpected deepening and widening of her own life experience. It had even drawn her into hitherto totally unexplored territory, as when she was asked, as a result of contacts made in the bureau, to teach English to three Sikh women from the Asian community, a mother and two daughters.

It seems that those who follow this path of self-giving in later years often find it leads into new areas. So it is with the last of these cases, a retired accountant who began, almost by accident, a scheme for organizing free transport for the elderly. It started simply enough by arranging a rota of volunteers to drive them to church. Soon he found himself drawn into trying to provide transport for a group who were stranded from shops and other facilities by the withdrawal of a bus service. So he became the organizer of a community mini-bus facility, and often the driver of it. He said, 'It's not just a matter of being kept busy. I can manage that in plenty of other ways, if I want to. What has really changed things for me is to find so many people dependent on me for what I can do for them. It's so different a life that sometimes I find it quite difficult to remember my former one.'

Realizing our limitations

It is largely a matter of common sense to recogize our limitations. We are not going to be in the full tide of youth by the time this challenge of making a new life reaches us, so we cannot expect to approach it with the same vigour or without evidence of physical wear and tear. The retired editor got it right when he said, 'One gets slower in thought and movement. But these are problems of advancing years, not of retirement. We all have to adjust to the running down process.' This seems obvious, yet it worries some people more than it should.

But the facts are encouraging. One is that modern medicine has dramatically changed the physical quality of life for those in later years. A fuller and more active life than ever before is now within their reach. 'The days of our age,' the Bible says, 'are threescore years and ten, and though men be so strong that they come to fourscore years, yet is their strength but labour and sorrow' (see Psalm 90:10). This is no longer generally true. On the other hand, the same Bible does say, 'To everything there is a season, and a time for every purpose under the sun... a time to get and a time to lose; a time to keep, and a time to cast away' (Ecclesiastes 3:1,6).

So the aches and pains of age, though nowadays much deferred, are still facts of life, and the limitations arising from them need to be duly recognized. It is therefore wise to bear them in mind when planning for a new life. In certainly two of the case histories related above, those concerned had to cope with some physical problems. The editor had difficulties with his eyes, and the woman executive had a serious illness shortly before her retirement. Part of their success in creating their new lives came through overcoming these difficulties.

Cultivating an inner life

The fourth step towards creating a new life in later years is to cultivate an inner life. It is by no means obligatory, and no such claim is made for it. Some may find it enough to have achieved satisfactory personal arrangements of their affairs, like the admirable people in those case histories, and to leave it at that. After all, it is not obligatory to find time for listening to fine music, but it is vastly rewarding, and that claim is certainly made for the cultivating of the inner life.

It is looking for meaning and purpose in what we do and are; and the later years of life offer a wonderful opportunity for sitting back and thinking about these fundamentals.

The temptation to look back over the years and wonder what on earth they have been about, with all their tensions and efforts, can be depressing. It is easy, in bad times, to conclude that they have been rather pointless, 'full of sound and fury, signifying nothing'. That kind of depression needs to be resisted, common though it is. It can be powerfully resisted by setting up a way of looking at things which finds satisfaction in something other than the entirely material aspects of daily life, like the daily stream of events in the world, its politics, its happenings, its gossip, its wars, its crises, which use up so much of our time. And never more so than now, when the media are all-invasive.

John Bunyan in *Pilgrim's Progress* gives a good picture of our modern situation. This is the Man with the Muckrake 'who could not look upward, but spent his time raking together the rubbish and dust on the floor of his room'. When Christian, who was being shown round the world of Vanity Fair, asked for an explanation of this odd sight, his guide said 'it was to show that Heaven is but a fable to some, and that things here are counted the only ones substantial. The man can look no way but downward. It is to show that earthly things, when they are with power upon men's minds, quite carry their hearts from God.'

We need an antidote to that kind of attitude today, just as much as in Bunyan's time, because it is so debilitating and boring and obscures so many wonderful things that are in our world, if only we could see them. An antidote used in all ages of human experience by those seeking to get away from the material aspects of the world for a while is the cultivation of the inner life. In essence, this is seeking to realize, and to exercise, the sense of eternal things within ourselves. All religions have recognized the importance of this. For Christians, the words of Jesus are of immense significance: 'The kingdom of God is within you.' That sums it up. Getting into this kingdom is by paths well attested and quite easy to follow, given persistence. They include a daily time of quiet for thought, reading and meditation. This outwardly simple habit can work wonders, bringing a new outlook on things often taken for granted and therefore not as valued as they might be.

The cultivation of what has been called, rather beautifully, 'the garden of the soul' can produce some lovely flowers. One of them is the gift of being suddenly able to see the extraordinary in the ordinary. A glimpse of grandchildren, for instance, when we are in a reflective and receptive state of mind, may bring more than the sight of their familiar little faces. It may also lead to a glimpse of the wonder of life, with its mysterious pattern of the succeeding generations, and of the love and kindness we may offer to these young people. Such thoughts can be 'too deep for words', and they can bring much joy.

There is another way in which this new sort of insight can work. It can enable us to know when, faced with some choice between right and wrong, we have done the right thing. There is a dramatic illustration of this in Tolstoy's novel, *Resurrection*. Nekhlyudov, the principal character, repenting of his dissolute life, resolves to befriend a prostitute he has been abusing. Following this resolution, outward things begin to look strangely different. He is in a country house. 'He went to the window and opened it. It was a moonlit night, quiet and fresh. The shadow of a poplar tree lay on the ground, making patterns. He drank in the air, cool and fresh. "God, how delightful," he said, meaning what was going on in his soul.' These strange moments are within reach of us all, if we give them a chance to come through.

It is true that this takes us a long way from the usual mundane concerns of later life. One woman commented that such concerns are too often exclusively material. She had recently been to a retirement conference and had noted the variety of speakers, all of whom showed the same characteristics.

A doctor talked about health, someone from the Inland Revenue talked about tax, someone talking on home hygiene mentioned the desirability of having handles on baths. There was even someone talking about yoga. She said, 'I didn't think this was good enough. We need to be thinking about other things in life than those. We need to be encouraged to think a bit on such big questions as what we are about, why we are here and where we are going.'

This approach may seem at first off-putting. But it need not be so. Certainly, people can cultivate their inner life in many ways, especially in the service of others. That indeed is the second of Christ's commandments. But the first is to worship God, in the sense of finding time and space for him in the inner life. And that is an important part in the search for meaning in what we are about, and why we are here.

How do we go about it? Let's start with a question: how much time do you give to the paper, or the news, and the like? Would you be prepared to set aside the same amount of time, or even half of it, daily, to a private exercise which begins by making a time of quiet and relaxation, both physical and mental? It might be easier for some in the morning, for others at night. The basic need is to draw the mind right back from everyday concerns. This is not easy; but practice can make it so, as many have found. There is nothing new about any of this.

Saintly people have tried it, ordinary people have tried it; the records they have left show it works. Mental and physical combine together here. Some psychotherapists or clinical psychologists give patients a tape to play at home to help them get into the right frame of mind for relaxation. The instructions given are often uncannily like those used by spiritual directors, the only difference being that the one is trying to help people think about themselves, while the other is trying to help them think about God.

Here is what one such tape advises. Place the body in a posture of ease, sitting or lying. Shut the doors, draw the curtains. If you wear glasses, take them off. Then relax the parts of the body, one by one: arms, neck, upper leg, lower leg, and so on. Take time over it. Then turn off your worries, one by one, money worries, health worries, relationship worries, and so on. Just so did St Anselm advise, centuries ago: 'Enter into the inner chamber of your soul and mind, shut out all things save God, and having barred the door, seek him.' The early stages can seem strange. But once the decision has been made to set aside a little time to this interval of quiet, it is possible that another voice will begin to be heard.

Here is a personal testimony to the truth of this from a man who has practised this sort of exercise for many years, and still does. Now in his seventies, he is a person with a very busy life behind him. He retired more than a decade ago from a position of some importance in the communications industry, has not missed that life, although he has made a new one, of which inner development has been an interesting and rewarding part. It started with the usual discovery of a sudden, unexpected amount of time at his disposal. Part of this time he devoted, quite early on, to a daily quiet time.

From the first he found that once outer noises had been shut out, another kind of sound began to be heard. He calls it, because that is his sort of background, 'the still small voice of God', thus quoting the Bible, a book familiar to him since his youth. Then he found that thinking of other people and their needs seemed to come naturally into the quiet. This deliberate thinking of other people and their concerns led on quite naturally to wondering how he could be of help to any of them who happened to be in need, the ill, the worried, especially the lonely, and this often became the starting point of action on their behalf.

He set aside the rest of this time of quiet to a planned programme of thoughtful reading and study. He would be the first to say that this sounds too pretentious as a description of what he was trying to do. Yet it proved, and again still does, to be richly rewarding. The principle at the core of it was not to allow anything into this space of his time which was only of passing interest, such as the news of the day, however important. His aim was to enrich his mental diet with more nourishing elements, drawing for it upon the huge treasures of world literature, by having on the go at any one time a book which was challenging to the mind, and which opened new areas of experience in understanding something of what great minds had said and notable people had experienced. (The editor mentioned earlier, incidentally, did exactly the same thing. He said he looked upon a time of quiet in his retirement days as a chance to read all the books he had always wanted to read, but never had.)

Interestingly, it became clear to the man we are thinking of now that it helped to have in mind some sort of standard for general outlook and conduct, if only to be able to pass it on to others as something worth knowing about. This was, and is, his guideline. Characteristically, he drew it from the Bible. 'All that is true, all that is noble, all that is just and pure, all that is lovable and gracious, whatever is excellent and admirable, fill all your heart with these things.' That advice from St Paul's letter to the Philippians he found wore well.

Without being at all judgmental of the lives of others, it proved useful in checking up on his own. From that developed a new habit. It started with the thought that if the bank could issue a monthly statement, it might be an idea to make one based on the debit or credit state of his personal account. So, using that passage from Paul's letter, he thought up this form of self-assessment.

A personal check-up

Have any of my actions recently measured up at all to the ideal of being 'excellent and admirable'?

Does it matter either way?
If not, why not?

What acts of kindness have I managed to do, especially when I didn't feel like it?

How often have I failed in patience with people who got on my nerves?

How much personal service have I given to neighbours and community lately?

How have I reacted, in my own mind, to any news story or media feature which seemed to clash with the ideals in the guideline passage? Indifferently or indignantly? Have I been happy or miserable since my last check-up? If the latter, why?

Have I managed to be grateful for any opportunities of service to others which have come my way?

In this way, this now elderly man has built up a fruitful habit of daily quiet, whenever possible, throughout his retirement years. It should be said, in fairness to him, that he is the least judgmental or outwardly moralistic of men. But he is a happy man. Others, with differing backgrounds and interests, may find quite different ways of building up their lives, or of finding standards to live by. But it does seem clear, from all the evidence, that this part of making a new life in later years is important, and can be very rewarding.

But how does this sort of thing, combined with an active looking out for opportunities of service to others, help the search for meaning in life? The answer is simple: it provides motive and purpose, which are essential to any meaningful living. It also provides an attractive pattern to daily habits. There is an importance in knowing what we are going to do, and when, and a sound private discipline recognizes this truth. In a sense, it is a way of keeping fit and in training for the useful things which, as senior people, we have to offer to the life of our times: experience, a certain amount of acquired wisdom, and, without being at all priggish about it, an example in decent standards of decent living. This is very valuable, especially to young people in these times of the privatization of morality when it is often difficult for them to find their way.

It was well put in a recent magazine article about older persons and their place in the scheme of things: 'We all know those among them who are giving far more to the community than they will ever receive. They are helping to sort the problems of others and adding to the well-being of society by their words and deeds; by their patience, cheerfulness, experience, understanding and listening!' To be able to offer any of those is to have purpose in life, and to be well on the way to finding meaning in it.

It needs to be said, though, that not many of these ends—motive and purpose, and the helpful actions which can follow—are likely to be achieved by living a private life in isolation from others. Keeping oneself to oneself won't work here. There is a story that John Wesley was challenged, after a meeting, by a man who claimed that a person's religion was his own business and nobody else's. Wesley's reply was: 'There is no such thing as a solitary Christian.' He might with equal truth have said that there is no such thing as a solitary man or woman who wants to find a full life of use to themselves and others. Solitariness is the path to loneliness, and a sad one it is.

Loneliness affects more people nowadays than ever before, being often a consequence of social changes. Feelings of belonging to a place and of having neighbours in it tend to fade when people are more mobile. So many move away after a comparatively short stay in one place, or go to some place where they are not known, like that factory foreman in Alan Bennett's play, who retired to the seaside and died of it. There is an increasing amount of sheer loneliness, and it affects the single even more than the married. Lonely people are the lost souls of our contemporary world, and there is a vast opportunity for service in trying to help them, which can often enough be done by simply offering them some of the time which later life gives us.

Any attempt to get into the life of the community requires the initial step of becoming involved. It is noticeable that each of the four people mentioned earlier did so. It is not a difficult thing to do. The world is full of people and organizations crying out for help. A call to any local voluntary service can open many doors to opportunities of service. Involvement in the life of a church can do the same but on a more personal level because it is joining in a family life of people sharing a common faith and outlook. Certainly, many good works are done under secular banners; but the church does present a way of consciously dedicating what we do as our personal service to God. What we do, or are invited to do, is not likely to be glamorous, but it is very likely to be rewarding, and stimulating, as well as an adventure in faith. Any church rich in people giving personal service in various forms—and there are few places which do not have several—demonstrates how effective such a fellowship can be, and how sound a move it can be to become a member of one.

One thing is for sure: it is not years that make people grow old before their time, but having nothing to love, nothing to hope for. Service of others in any form, and under any banner, is a way out of the one-way street of service of self alone. It has been well said that we die only when we fail to take root in other people's lives.

Summing it all up

Those four steps we started with are useful in shaping a good attitude to making a new life in later years, and can be seen in practice to work well. Others have found them so, and had things to say about them. Some are worth noting. Shakespeare had a word about getting rid of the past in the Prologue to *The Tempest*:

> 'What's past is prologue,
> what's to come
> is yours and my discharge.'

Our second step, filling the future with meaningful activity, really means the right use of time, and so arranging life that we have much to do in it. Winifred Holtby, who wrote in the early 1920s, had a good word about this:

> 'God give me work till my life shall end, and life till my work is done.'

Then we need to realize our limitations, certainly. But let's not overdo it. Be as old as we feel but not feel older than we are. Bernard Baruch, quoted in a Sayings of the Week feature some time ago, got it about right: 'I will never be an old man. To me, old age is always fifteen years older than I am.'

Finally, give a bit of time to quiet and thought. What about? This world, and the one to come. An old piece of verse by Longfellow sums up this and everything else rather well:

'What then?
Shall we sit idly down and say,
The night has come; it is no longer day?
For age is opportunity, no less
Than youth itself,
though in another dress.
And as the evening twilight fades away,
The sky is filled with stars,
invisible by day.'